THE

NITRIC OXIDE

DIET

COOKBOOK

SARAH JACK

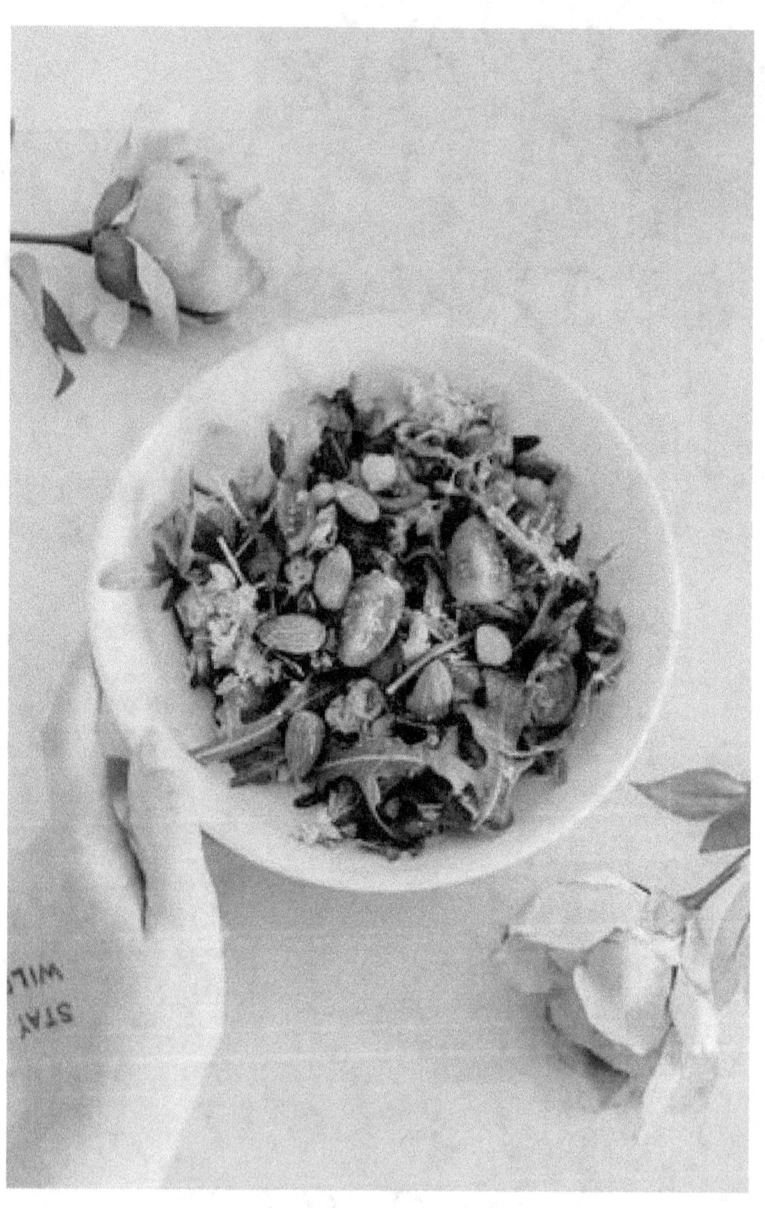

STAY
WILD

COPYRIGHT

TABLE OF CONTENTS

Table of Contents

INTRODUCTION

The chemical nitric oxide (NO) is essential to many physiological processes in both the human body and other animals. It has the chemical formula NO and is an odorless, colorless gas made up of one nitrogen (N) and one oxygen (O) atom. Nitric oxide's main characteristics are as follows:

1. Nitric oxide is a signaling molecule that also functions as a vasodilator, relaxing and enlarging blood vessels. This characteristic is crucial for controlling blood pressure and preserving healthy blood flow.

2. Nitric oxide is created in the body by nitric oxide synthase (NOS) enzymes, which convert the amino acid L-arginine into NO through an enzymatic process. Neuronal NOS (nNOS or NOS1), inducible NOS (iNOS or NOS2), and endothelial NOS (eNOS or NOS3) are the three isoforms of NOS. Each isoform is expressed in various tissues and has a particular purpose.

3. Functions in the Body:

- Vasodilation: NO causes the smooth muscles that line blood vessels to relax, which increases blood flow. This is crucial for controlling blood pressure and making sure that tissues receive enough oxygen and nutrients.

- NO functions as a neurotransmitter in the neurological system, assisting in the signaling between nerve cells.

- immunological Response: NO from iNOS contributes to the immunological response, assisting in the fight against infections and inflammation.

- Cell Signaling: NO engages in a number of cell signaling pathways that control activities such as apoptosis (cell death) and gene expression.

- Male erectile dysfunction: In order to enhance blood flow, relax the blood vessels in the penis, and start and maintain an erection, NO is essential.

4. Nitric oxide is employed in medical applications because of its role in vasodilation and effects on the cardiovascular system. Adults with acute respiratory distress syndrome (ARDS) and babies with chronic pulmonary hypertension both occasionally receive treatment with inhaled nitric oxide.

5. Dietary Nitric Oxide: The body can produce NO in part from dietary sources of nitric oxide precursors like nitrate and nitrite, which are present in foods like leafy greens and beets. Under various circumstances, most notably in the presence of acidic stomach conditions, these chemicals are transformed into NO.

6. In the same way as carbon monoxide (CO) and hydrogen sulfide (H2S), nitric oxide is regarded as a signaling gas. These tiny gas molecules are crucial for cell signaling and the control of several physiological processes.

7. Nitric oxide supplements: In an effort to boost NO production and improve blood flow, some athletes and anyone interested in improving sports performance have utilized nitric oxide supplements, frequently containing substances like L-arginine. The efficacy of these supplements is up for debate, so it's important to carefully assess both their safety and efficacy.

Nitric oxide is a crucial chemical that regulates a variety of bodily processes, including blood flow, neurotransmission, immunological response, and more. It is a topic of continuous study and clinical interest because to its significance in a number of physiological processes.

LIFESTYLE HABITS FOR NITRIC OXIDE BOOSTING

Nitric oxide (NO) is a crucial signaling molecule in the body with a wide array of physiological functions, including the regulation of blood flow, immune response, and neurotransmission. Its impact on cardiovascular health, in particular, has garnered significant attention. Beyond dietary considerations, adopting specific lifestyle habits can contribute to the natural production and optimization of nitric oxide levels, promoting overall well-being. In this exploration, we delve into lifestyle habits that play a pivotal role in boosting nitric oxide.

- **Regular Exercise and Physical Activity:**

Physical activity stands as a cornerstone in the lifestyle habits that support nitric oxide production. Exercise induces the release of endothelial nitric oxide, improving blood vessel function and promoting vasodilation. Both aerobic exercises, such as running or cycling, and resistance training have shown positive effects on nitric oxide levels. Engaging in regular physical activity not only enhances cardiovascular health but also fosters an environment conducive to optimal nitric oxide synthesis.

- **Sun Exposure and Vitamin D:**

Sunlight exposure is not only essential for vitamin D synthesis but also influences nitric oxide production. When the skin is exposed to sunlight, it triggers the conversion of nitrate stored in the skin to nitric oxide. Vitamin D, synthesized in response to sunlight exposure, further contributes to endothelial function. Striking a balance between sun safety and moderate exposure can be beneficial for both vitamin D levels and nitric oxide production.

- **Stress Management and Relaxation Techniques:**

Chronic stress has been linked to impaired endothelial function and decreased nitric oxide bioavailability. Incorporating stress management techniques, such as meditation, deep breathing exercises, or yoga, can positively influence nitric oxide levels. These practices contribute to a reduction in stress hormones, creating an environment that supports the healthy functioning of blood vessels.

- **Quality Sleep:**

Adequate and quality sleep is a crucial aspect of overall well-being, and its influence extends to nitric oxide regulation. Studies have shown that insufficient or poor-quality sleep can negatively impact endothelial function and nitric oxide production. Establishing a consistent sleep routine, creating a conducive sleep environment, and addressing sleep disorders can contribute to improved nitric oxide levels.

- **Hydration and Nitrate-Rich Foods:**

Proper hydration is fundamental for the body's biochemical processes, including the conversion of nitrate to nitric oxide. Nitrate-rich foods, such as leafy greens and beets, are a valuable dietary source. These foods contain inorganic nitrate, which, through a series of biological processes, can be converted to nitric oxide. Staying well-hydrated supports these conversion pathways and ensures the availability of nitrate for nitric oxide synthesis.

- **Balanced Nutrition:**

Beyond nitrate-rich foods, adopting a balanced and nutritious diet contributes to overall cardiovascular health and, subsequently, nitric oxide production. Nutrients such as antioxidants, vitamins, and minerals play supportive roles in maintaining the health of the endothelium, the inner lining of blood vessels where nitric oxide is produced. Including a variety of fruits, vegetables, whole grains, and lean proteins in the diet provides essential nutrients that foster optimal nitric oxide function.

- **Limiting Tobacco and Alcohol Consumption:**

Tobacco smoke contains harmful chemicals that can damage the endothelium and reduce nitric oxide availability. Quitting smoking or avoiding exposure to secondhand smoke is a crucial step in supporting cardiovascular health. Similarly, excessive alcohol consumption can have detrimental effects on the cardiovascular system. Moderation or abstinence from alcohol contributes to a healthier endothelial environment and, consequently, enhanced nitric oxide production.

- **Maintaining a Healthy Body Weight:**

Obesity is associated with endothelial dysfunction and decreased nitric oxide bioavailability. Adopting a lifestyle that includes regular physical activity and a balanced diet contributes to maintaining a healthy body weight. Weight management, along with other lifestyle habits, creates a favorable environment for nitric oxide synthesis, promoting cardiovascular health.

- **Conclusion:**

In the intricate interplay of physiological processes, lifestyle habits emerge as influential factors in the regulation of nitric oxide. These habits not only support cardiovascular health but also contribute to the broader landscape of overall well-being. Regular exercise, sunlight exposure, stress management, quality sleep, hydration, balanced nutrition, and healthy lifestyle choices collectively create an environment that fosters optimal nitric oxide production.

As individuals embark on the journey of cultivating these lifestyle habits, they lay the foundation for a healthier cardiovascular system and, by extension, a healthier life. Nitric oxide, with its far-reaching effects, becomes a marker of the intricate dance between our choices and the physiological responses that shape our well-being. It is a reminder that beyond pharmaceutical interventions, the power to enhance health often lies in the daily choices we make to support the body's natural mechanisms.

NITRIC OXIDE DIET

A "nitrate-rich diet," also known as a "nitric oxide diet," emphasizes the consumption of foods with a high nitrate content. Foods high in nitrate are thought to increase the body's synthesis of nitric oxide (NO), which has a number of health advantages, especially for cardiovascular health and exercise capacity. An essential component of a nitric oxide diet is as follows:

1. Nitrate-Rich Foods: Foods that are naturally high in nitrates are prioritized in a nitric oxide diet. These foods consist of:

Leafy greens: Swiss chard, kale, spinach, and arugula are all great sources of nitrates.

Beets: The high nitrate content of beets and beetroot juice is widely recognized.

Radishes: Some radishes, such as daikon radishes, are excellent suppliers of nitrates.

Another vegetable that contains nitrates is celery.

Carrots: Carrots have a moderate nitrate content as well.

2. Nitrate Conversion to Nitric Oxide: The body can convert nitrates from these foods to nitric oxide (NO) through a number of biochemical processes, especially in the mouth and digestive system. Dietary nitrates are metabolized by oral bacteria into nitrites, which are then transformed into NO in the stomach and bloodstream.

3. Health Advantages: Eating a diet high in nitrates may provide the following advantages:

- Nitric oxide is a vasodilator, which means that it relaxes blood vessels, which improves blood flow and may result in a drop in blood pressure.

- Improved Exercise Performance: Some athletes and fitness enthusiasts think that by boosting the amount of oxygen delivered to muscles, a nitrate-rich diet may enhance endurance and exercise performance.

- Cardiovascular Health: By assisting in the maintenance of healthy blood pressure and lowering the risk of heart disease, increased nitric oxide generation may have a good effect on cardiovascular health.

4. Other Sources of Nitrate: Nitrates can also be present in trace amounts in some fruits, cereals, and processed foods in addition to vegetables. However, a nitric oxide diet places a lot of emphasis on nitrates found in naturally occurring, unprocessed foods like leafy greens and beets.

5. Factors: Although a nitric oxide diet may have certain advantages, it's important to take into account each person's dietary choices, total nutritional requirements, and any pre-existing medical issues. Before making any dietary changes, it's a good idea to speak with a healthcare provider or a qualified

dietitian if you have any particular health issues or dietary limitations.

6. Balanced Diet: A nitric oxide diet need to be a component of a well-rounded and diverse diet. While nitrate-rich foods are advantageous, to ensure enough nutrition overall, they should be included in a diet that also contains a variety of nutrients from fruits, vegetables, whole grains, lean proteins, and healthy fats.

In conclusion, a nitric oxide diet emphasizes the consumption of foods high in nitrates to encourage the body's generation of nitric oxide, which may improve cardiovascular health and athletic performance. It can be good to include nitrate-rich vegetables like leafy greens and beets in your diet, but in order to achieve your nutritional needs, it's crucial to keep an overall diet in balance.

BENEFITS OF NITRIC OXIDE DIET

A diet heavy in nitrate-rich foods and other foods that promote nitric oxide (NO) may have various positive effects on one's general health and wellbeing. The following are some of the main advantages of a nitric oxide diet:

1. Better Cardiovascular Health:

* Vasodilation: Nitric oxide relaxes and expands blood vessels since it is a potent vasodilator. This result contributes to better blood flow, lowered blood pressure, and improved cardiovascular health. All body parts, including the heart and brain, need healthy blood flow to receive oxygen and nutrients.

* Blood pressure Control: Better blood pressure control may be facilitated by increased nitric oxide synthesis, which may lower the risk of hypertension (high blood pressure) and associated cardiovascular diseases.

2. Improved Physical Performance:

- Nitric oxide aids in blood artery dilation, which increases the amount of oxygen-rich blood that can reach muscles during activity. Performance during exercise and endurance can both be improved by this better oxygen delivery.

- Delayed exhaustion: According to some research, eating foods high in nitrates may help people exercise longer and maybe at higher intensities by delaying the onset of exhaustion during physical activity.

3. Enhancement of Endothelial Function:

- Endothelial cells line the interior of blood arteries and are essential for controlling blood coagulation and vascular tone. In order to maintain proper endothelial function, which is crucial for overall vascular health, nitric oxide is produced.

4. Reduced Inflammation:

- Nitric oxide contains anti-inflammatory qualities that can help lessen tissue and blood vessel inflammation. Cardiovascular disease and other health problems, including chronic inflammation, are linked.

5. Enhanced Cognitive Performance:

- Nitric oxide may help to improve memory and mental clarity by increasing blood flow to the brain and oxygen supply to the area.

6. Possible Decrease in Risk Factors:

- A diet high in nitric oxide may help reduce some heart disease risk factors such high blood pressure, high cholesterol, and arterial stiffness.

7. Effects of antioxidants:

- Even nitric oxide itself has antioxidant properties that can assist the body fight off dangerous free radicals. This antioxidant quality can help protect against oxidative stress and improve general health.

8. Dietary Diversity:

- Several nitrate-rich fruits and vegetables that are high in necessary vitamins, minerals, and dietary fiber are encouraged as part of a nitric oxide diet. This supports a balanced diet and encourages overall nutritional diversity.

The nitric oxide diet should be a part of a comprehensive healthy eating plan, despite the fact that it may provide these potential advantages. Maintaining good health also requires balance and moderation in your nutrition, frequent exercise, and other aspects of your lifestyle.

Before making any dietary changes, it is advised to speak with a healthcare provider or registered dietitian who can offer individualized counsel and suggestions catered to your particular requirements and goals. This is especially important if you have any particular health conditions or concerns.

EXERCISE AND NITRIC OXIDE

Exercise, often hailed as a cornerstone of a healthy lifestyle, extends its influence far beyond the realms of weight management and muscular strength. One of the fascinating intersections within the intricate web of physiological responses to exercise involves nitric oxide (NO). This tiny molecule, produced within the body, plays a pivotal role in cardiovascular health and is profoundly influenced by regular physical activity. Delve into the symbiotic relationship between exercise and nitric oxide, uncovering the mechanisms, benefits, and implications for overall well-being.

- **Exercise as a Catalyst for Nitric Oxide Production:**

The connection between exercise and nitric oxide lies in the dynamic interplay between mechanical forces and biochemical responses within the vascular system. As muscles contract during physical activity, especially aerobic exercises like running, cycling, or swimming, shear stress is exerted on the endothelial cells lining the blood vessels. This shear stress acts as a trigger for the release of nitric oxide.

During exercise, the increased blood flow and shear stress stimulate the enzyme endothelial nitric oxide synthase (eNOS) to produce nitric oxide. This process is particularly vital because the enhanced blood flow necessitates greater oxygen delivery to working muscles.

Nitric oxide ensures that blood vessels expand to accommodate this increased demand, facilitating optimal oxygen and nutrient transport to active tissues.

- **Types of Exercise and Their Impact on Nitric Oxide:**

Aerobic Exercise:

Aerobic or endurance exercises, characterized by sustained periods of moderate-intensity activity, have been extensively studied for their positive effects on nitric oxide production. The rhythmic and repetitive nature of activities like jogging or cycling enhances endothelial function and promotes the sustained release of nitric oxide.

Resistance Training:

While aerobic exercise has been a focal point in nitric oxide research, resistance training also demonstrates its influence. Resistance exercises, including weight lifting and strength training, induce a transient increase in blood pressure. This acute pressure change contributes to the release of nitric oxide, supporting vasodilation and maintaining blood flow to the working muscles.

Interval Training:

High-intensity interval training (HIIT), characterized by alternating short bursts of intense exercise with periods of rest or lower-intensity activity, has gained popularity for its efficiency in improving cardiovascular fitness. Studies suggest that HIIT may have favorable effects on nitric oxide levels, contributing to cardiovascular health benefits.

- **Nitric Oxide Benefits Amplified by Exercise:**

Improved Blood Flow:

The vasodilatory effect of nitric oxide induced by exercise translates into enhanced blood flow. This is particularly significant for cardiovascular health as it improves the delivery of oxygen and nutrients to various tissues, supporting overall physiological function.

Blood Pressure Regulation:

Nitric oxide's role in vasodilation helps regulate blood pressure. Exercise-induced nitric oxide production contributes to maintaining healthy blood pressure levels, reducing the risk of hypertension and related cardiovascular issues.

Endothelial Health:

Regular exercise promotes the health and function of endothelial cells. The endothelium serves as the site of nitric oxide production, and exercise helps maintain its integrity, ensuring optimal nitric oxide synthesis.

Anti-Inflammatory Effects:

Nitric oxide exhibits anti-inflammatory properties, and exercise further contributes to a reduction in chronic inflammation. This dual impact supports cardiovascular health by mitigating inflammatory factors that contribute to atherosclerosis and other cardiovascular diseases.

Enhanced Exercise Performance:

The improved blood flow and oxygen delivery facilitated by nitric oxide play a crucial role in exercise performance. Athletes and fitness enthusiasts may experience enhanced endurance and reduced fatigue due to optimized circulation.

- **Implications for Cardiovascular Health:**

Prevention of Atherosclerosis:

Atherosclerosis, the buildup of plaque in the arteries, is a leading cause of cardiovascular diseases. Nitric oxide's vasodilatory effects help prevent the development of atherosclerotic plaques, reducing the risk of conditions like coronary artery disease.

Management of Hypertension:

Hypertension, or high blood pressure, is a significant risk factor for cardiovascular events. Exercise-induced nitric oxide production contributes to blood pressure regulation, making regular physical activity an integral component of hypertension management.

Reduced Risk of Cardiovascular Events:

The combination of improved blood flow, blood pressure regulation, and anti-inflammatory effects contributes to an overall reduction in the risk of cardiovascular events such as heart attacks and strokes.

- **Practical Recommendations:**

Consistent Exercise Routine:

Engaging in regular physical activity is key to unlocking the benefits of exercise-induced nitric oxide production. Aim for at least 150 minutes of moderate-intensity aerobic exercise or 75 minutes of vigorous-intensity aerobic exercise per week, combined with resistance training twice a week.

Variety in Exercise Modalities:

Incorporate a mix of aerobic exercises, resistance training, and potentially interval training to ensure a comprehensive impact on nitric oxide production. Variety not only prevents monotony but also engages different physiological pathways.

Individualized Approach:

Recognize that individual responses to exercise can vary. Factors such as age, fitness level, and health conditions influence the body's capacity to produce nitric oxide. Tailor exercise routines to individual capabilities and consult with healthcare professionals when needed.

- **Conclusion:**

The symbiotic relationship between exercise and nitric oxide underscores the profound impact of lifestyle choices on cardiovascular health. Regular physical activity emerges as a potent catalyst for nitric oxide production, contributing to vasodilation, blood flow optimization, and overall cardiovascular well-being. As individuals commit to a lifestyle that embraces exercise, they embark on a journey towards a healthier heart, reduced cardiovascular risks, and an improved quality of life. The integration of exercise into daily routines becomes a proactive and empowering step toward cardiovascular health, fueled by the symbiotic dance between the body's dynamic response to movement and the cardiovascular benefits bestowed by nitric oxide.

NITRIC OXIDE DIET RECIPES

Beet and Spinach Salad

Ingredients:

- 2 medium beets, roasted and chopped,

- 4 cups fresh leaves of spinach

- Chopped walnuts, 1/4 cup

- 1/4 cup crumbled feta cheese

- Balsamic vinaigrette dressing

Instructions:

- Peel and dice the beets after baking them in the oven until they are soft.

- In a big bowl, combine the spinach, chopped beets, walnuts, and feta cheese.

- Add balsamic vinaigrette dressing and blend by drizzling it over the salad. Serve as a nutritious salad.

Beet and Berry Smoothie

Ingredients:

- 1 small beet, cooked and peeled

- 1 cup of mixed berries, such as raspberries, blueberries, and strawberries

- Half a banana

- Spinach leaves, 1 cup

- 1 cup of almond milk without sugar

- 1 tablespoon honey (optional)

Instructions:

- In a blender, mix each ingredient until it is completely smooth.

- If desired, use honey to adjust sweetness.

- Pour this nutrient-rich smoothie into a glass and savor it.

Grilled Salmon with Beet Salsa

Ingredients:

- 4 fillets of salmon

- chopped and boiled two medium beets

- 1/2 red onion, chopped finely

- 1/4 cup chopped fresh cilantro

- 1 lime's juice

- Pepper and salt as desired

Instructions:

- Cook the salmon fillets completely on the grill.

- To make the beet salsa, mix the chopped beets, red onion, cilantro, lime juice, salt, and pepper in a basin.

- Serve the salmon with the beet salsa on top.

Spinach and Beet Hummus

Ingredients:

- 1 cup cooked beets, diced

- Cooked chickpeas, 1 cup

- Fresh spinach greens, 2 cups

- Garlic cloves, two

- Juice of 1 lemon

- Tahini, 2 tablespoons

- Olive oil, two tablespoons

- Pepper and salt as desired

Instructions:

- In a food processor, mix beets, chickpeas, spinach, garlic, lemon juice, tahini, olive oil, salt, and pepper.

- Until smooth, blend.

- Serve as a dip with vegetables sticks or whole-grain crackers.

Quinoa and Beet Salad

Ingredients:

- 1 cup cooked and chilled quinoa

- 1/2 cucumber, diced

- 2 medium beets, roasted and diced

- 1/4 cup minced fresh parsley

- 1/4 cup crumbled goat cheese

- Lemon vinaigrette dressing

Instructions:

- Quinoa, diced cucumber, diced beets, parsley, and crumbled goat cheese should all be combined in a big bowl.

- Add a lemon vinaigrette dressing and combine thoroughly by tossing.

Beet and Carrot Soup

Ingredients:

- 4 medium beets, roasted and skinned

- 1 chopped onion

- 2 big carrots

- 4 cups of vegetable broth

- A half-cup of coconut milk (or a dairy-free substitute)

- Pepper and salt as desired

Instructions:

- Cook the onions and carrots in a big pot until they are tender.

- Add veggie broth and roasted beets. Simmer the carrots until they are soft.

- Pour the soup into an immersion blender and purée it.

- Add salt, pepper, and coconut milk by stirring. Serve after a gentle reheat.

Spinach and Beet Smoothie Bowl

Ingredients:

- 1 tiny beet, boiled and peeled

- Half a banana

- 1/2 cup Greek yogurt (or dairy-free alternative)

- Toppings include granola, banana slices, berries, and chia seeds.

Instructions:

- Banana, spinach, beet, and Greek yogurt should all be thoroughly blended.

- Pour into a bowl and top with your favorite toppings for a nutritious smoothie bowl.

Quiche with Beets and Feta

Ingredients:

- 1 pie crust, either homemade or purchased.

- 3 medium beets, roasted and sliced

- 1 cup crumbled feta cheese

- Four big eggs

- One cup of milk (or a dairy-free substitute)

- Pepper and salt as desired

Instructions:

- Set the oven's temperature to 375°F (190°C).

- Place the feta cheese crumbles and slices of roasted beets in the pie shell.

- Whisk the eggs, milk, salt, and pepper in another bowl.

- Over the beets and feta, pour the egg mixture.

- Bake the quiche for 35 to 40 minutes, or until it is set and the top is just beginning to brown.

Spinach and Beet Power Bowl

Ingredients:

- 2 cups cooked quinoa

- Fresh spinach greens, 2 cups

- 1 cooked and thinly sliced medium beet

- Cooked chickpeas, half a cup

- 1/4 cup pumpkin seeds

- Balsamic vinaigrette dressing

Instructions:

- Place cooked quinoa, fresh spinach, sliced beet, chickpeas, and pumpkin seeds in a large bowl.

- Add balsamic vinaigrette dressing and gently toss.

Beet and Orange Smoothie

Ingredients:

- 1 small beet, cooked and peeled

- 1 orange, peeled and segmented

- 1/2 banana

- Half a cup of Greek yogurt (or a dairy-free substitute)

- 1/2 cup of orange juice or water

- Honey or maple syrup (optional, for sweetness)

Instructions:

- To make a smooth mixture, combine the cooked beet, orange segments, banana, Greek yogurt, and water (or orange juice).

- Add honey or maple syrup if additional sweetness is desired.

- Serve as a refreshing beet and orange smoothie.

Watermelon and Beet Salad

Ingredients:

- 2 cups of chopped watermelon

- 2 medium beets, roasted and diced

- 1/4 cup crumbled feta cheese

- Fresh mint leaves

- Balsamic vinaigrette dressing

Instructions:

- In a bowl, mix roasted beets and diced watermelon.

- Add some feta cheese crumbles and fresh mint leaves as a garnish.

- Serve as a cooling salad with a balsamic vinaigrette dressing.

Beet and Spinach Stuffed Chicken Breast

Ingredients:

- 2 skinless, boneless chicken breasts

- 1 medium beet, diced after roasting

- Fresh spinach leaves, 1 cup

- 1/4 cup goat cheese

- Almond oil

- Pepper and salt as desired

Instructions:

- Set the oven's temperature to 375°F (190°C).

- To create a pocket, butterfly the chicken breasts.

- Each chicken breast should be stuffed with goat cheese, spinach, and sliced beets.

- Add salt and pepper to taste.

- The chicken should be seared on both sides in hot, medium-high olive oil.

- When the chicken is cooked through, transfer it to a baking sheet and bake for 20 to 25 minutes.

Beet and Blueberry Smoothie

Ingredients:

- 1 small beet, boiled and peeled

- 1/2 cup fresh or frozen blueberries

- Half a banana

- 1 cup dairy-free milk substitute (or unsweetened almond milk)

- Chia seeds, one tablespoon

- Honey or maple syrup (optional, for sweetness)

Instructions:

- Banana, almond milk, chia seeds, cooked beet, and blueberries should all be thoroughly blended.

- Add honey or maple syrup for sweetness if desired.

- Enjoy this colorful beet and blueberry smoothie by pouring it into a glass.

Spinach and Beet Quinoa Bowl

Ingredients:

- One cup of cooked quinoa

- Fresh spinach greens, 2 cups

- 1 medium beet, roasted and sliced

- 1/2 avocado, sliced

- 1/4 cup crumbled feta cheese

- Lemon-tahini dressing

Instructions:

- Place cooked quinoa, spinach, roasted beet pieces, avocado, and feta cheese crumbles in a bowl.

- Add the lemon-tahini dressing and gently stir.

Beet and Lentil Soup

Ingredients:

- 2 medium beets, roasted and chopped

- Red lentils, 1 cup

- One sliced onion

- 2 minced garlic cloves

- Six cups of vegetable stock

- 1 teaspoon cumin

- Pepper and salt as desired

Instructions:

- Sauté the onions and garlic in a big pot until they are tender.

- Beets, red lentils, cumin, vegetable broth, salt, and pepper should all be added.

- Lentils should be simmered until they are soft and the soup is thick.

- Serve as a filling and healthy lentil and beet soup.

Spinach and Beet Smoothie with Chia Seeds

Ingredients:

- 1 small beet, cooked and peeled

- fresh spinach leaves, 2 cups

- Greek yogurt, or a dairy-free substitute, in 1/2 cup

- Chia seeds, one tablespoon

- 1/2 cup dairy-free milk (or unsweetened almond milk)

- Honey or maple syrup (optional, for sweetness)

Instructions:

- Greek yogurt, fresh spinach, chia seeds, and almond milk should all be thoroughly blended.

- Add honey or maple syrup for sweetness if desired.

- Pour this healthy smoothie into a glass, and savor it.

Roasted Beet and Goat Cheese Crostini

Ingredients:

- 2 medium beets, roasted and sliced

- Goat cheese

- Fresh thyme leaves

- Olive oil

- Balsamic glaze (optional)

Instructions:

- Slices of baguette can be grilled or baked.

- Each slice should have goat cheese on it.

- Add fresh thyme leaves and slices of roasted beet on top.

- Drizzle with olive oil and balsamic glaze if desired. Serve as an appetizer.

Beet and Arugula Pizza

Ingredients:

- Pizza dough (either homemade or from a supermarket)

- Pesto or tomato sauce

- 2 medium beets, roasted and thinly sliced

- Fresh arugula leaves

- Mozzarella cheese or goat cheese

- Almond oil

Instructions:

- Roll out the pizza dough and preheat the oven.

- Over the dough, spread pesto or tomato sauce.

- Slices of cheese of your choosing should then be placed on top of the roasted beets.

- Bake according to the directions on the pizza dough.

- Top the dish with new arugula and a sprinkle of olive oil after it comes out of the oven.

Beet and Carrot Coleslaw

Ingredients:

- Grated beets from two medium-sized beets

- Grated two big carrots

- Greek yogurt, or a dairy-free substitute, in 1/2 cup

- Apple cider vinegar, 2 tablespoons

- 1 tablespoon of maple syrup or honey

- Pepper and salt as desired

Instructions:

- Combine grated carrots and beets in a big bowl.

- Greek yogurt, apple cider vinegar, honey or maple syrup, salt, and pepper should all be combined in a different bowl.

- Grate the vegetables, then add the dressing and stir to evenly coat.

- Before serving as a colorful coleslaw, place in the refrigerator for at least 30 minutes.

Spinach and Beet Risotto

Ingredients:

- 1 cup Arborio rice

- 2 medium beets, roasted and diced

- Fresh spinach greens, 2 cups

- A half-cup of grated Parmesan cheese (or a dairy-free substitute)

- 4 cups of veggie broth

- 1/2 cup dry white wine (optional)

- Almond oil

- Pepper and salt as desired

Instructions:

- Cook Arborio rice in olive oil in a big skillet till it turns translucent.

- Continue to sauté after adding the diced beets.

- If using, add white wine and simmer until it is absorbed.

- Vegetable broth should be added gradually, one ladle at a time, and stirred until absorbed before adding more.

- Add fresh spinach leaves and freshly grated Parmesan cheese to the rice once it is creamy and cooked to your preference.

- Season with salt and pepper and serve as a comforting beet and spinach risotto.

Beet and Spinach Breakfast Wrap

Ingredients:

- 1 whole-grain wrap or tortilla

- 1 cooked and sliced small beet

- Fresh spinach leaves, 1 cup

- 2 eggs (or tofu scramble for a vegan option)

- Feta cheese, if desired

- Pepper and salt as desired

Instructions:

- Scramble the eggs (or prepare tofu scramble).

- On the wrap, put the cooked eggs (or tofu).

- If preferred, garnish with thinly sliced beets, new spinach leaves, and feta cheese.

- Add salt and pepper, roll the wrap up, and eat as a filling breakfast.

Beet and Lentil Salad with Avocado

Ingredients:

- 2 medium beets, roasted and chopped

- Cooked green or brown lentils, 1 cup

- 1 diced avocado

- 1/4 cup coarsely chopped red onion

- Fresh leaves of cilantro

- Vinaigrette made with lime

Instructions:

- Beets, cooked lentils, diced avocado, and red onion are all combined in a bowl.

- Drizzle with lime vinaigrette dressing and toss to combine.

- Serve the beet and lentil salad with fresh cilantro leaves as garnish.

Beet and Berry Parfait

Ingredients:

- 1 small beet, cooked and peeled

- 1 cup mixed berries (e.g., strawberries, blueberries, raspberries)

- Greek yogurt (or dairy-free alternative)

- Granola

- Honey or maple syrup (optional, for sweetness)

Instructions:

- The cooked beet should be smoothed out.

- Greek yogurt, granola, mixed berries, and beet puree should be arranged in a glass or bowl.

- If desired, drizzle with honey or maple syrup.

- For a filling and eye-catching parfait, repeat the layers as desired.

Spinach and Beet Pesto Pasta

Ingredients:

- 8 oz whole-grain pasta (e.g., penne)

- 2 medium beets, roasted and diced

- 2 cups fresh spinach leaves

- 1/4 cup pine nuts

- 2 cloves garlic

- 1/2 cup grated Parmesan cheese (or dairy-free alternative)

- Olive oil

- Salt and pepper to taste

Instructions:

- Pasta should be prepared as directed on the package, drained, and then set aside.

- Diced beets, new spinach, pine nuts, garlic, and Parmesan cheese are combined in a food processor.

- Add olive oil in small amounts while the machine is running until the pesto is the right consistency.

- Combine the beet and spinach pesto with the cooked pasta. Before serving, season with salt and pepper.

Beet and Pineapple Smoothie Bowl

Ingredients:

- 1 small beet, cooked and peeled

- 1 cup pineapple chunks (fresh or frozen)

- 1/2 banana

- 1/2 cup coconut milk (or dairy-free alternative)

- Toppings: shredded coconut, sliced banana, chia seeds

Instructions:

- Banana, pineapple pieces, coconut milk, and cooked beet should all be thoroughly blended.

- A tropical beet and pineapple smoothie bowl can be made by pouring the smoothie into a bowl and adding your own garnishes.

Nitrate-Rich Green Smoothie

Ingredients:

- 1 cup spinach

- 1/2 cup kale

- 1/2 cup beetroot, chopped

- 1/2 cup cucumber, sliced

- 1 green apple, cored and chopped

- 1 tablespoon chia seeds

- 1 cup water or coconut water

Instructions:

- Combine all ingredients in a blender.

- Blend until smooth.

- Pour into a glass and enjoy.

Citrus Berry Blast Smoothie Bowl

Ingredients:

- 1 cup mixed berries (strawberries, blueberries, raspberries)

- 1/2 banana, frozen

- 1/2 cup Greek yogurt

- 1 tablespoon flaxseeds

- 1 tablespoon honey

Instructions:

- Blend berries, banana, Greek yogurt, and flaxseeds until smooth.

- Pour into a bowl and drizzle with honey.

Walnut and Spinach Pesto Pasta

Ingredients:

- 8 oz whole wheat pasta

- 2 cups spinach

- 1/2 cup walnuts

- 2 cloves garlic

- 1/2 cup Parmesan cheese, grated

- 1/2 cup olive oil

Instructions:

- Cook pasta according to package instructions.

- In a food processor, blend spinach, walnuts, garlic, and Parmesan.

- With the processor running, slowly add olive oil until smooth.

- Toss pesto with cooked pasta.

Grilled Salmon with Lemon-Dill Sauce

Ingredients:

- 4 salmon fillets

- 2 lemons, juiced

- 1 tablespoon fresh dill, chopped

- 2 cloves garlic, minced

- Salt and pepper to taste

Instructions:

- Preheat grill to medium-high heat.

- Season salmon with salt, pepper, and minced garlic.

- Grill salmon for 4-5 minutes per side.

- In a bowl, mix lemon juice and dill. Drizzle over grilled salmon.

Dark Chocolate Avocado Mousse

Ingredients:

- 2 ripe avocados

- 1/4 cup cocoa powder

- 1/4 cup maple syrup

- 1 teaspoon vanilla extract

- Pinch of salt

Instructions:

- Scoop avocados into a blender.

- Add cocoa powder, maple syrup, vanilla extract, and a pinch of salt.

- Blend until smooth and refrigerate before serving.

Nitrate-Packed Veggie Wrap

Ingredients:

- Whole grain wrap

- Hummus

- Spinach leaves

- Sliced cucumber

- Shredded carrots

- Sliced bell peppers

Instructions:

- Spread hummus on a whole grain wrap.

- Layer with spinach, cucumber, carrots, and bell peppers.

- Roll the wrap and slice into halves.

Roasted Beet and Goat Cheese Salad

Ingredients:

- Mixed greens

- 1 cup roasted beets, sliced

- 1/4 cup goat cheese, crumbled

- 1/4 cup walnuts, toasted

- Balsamic vinaigrette

Instructions:

- Arrange mixed greens on a plate.

- Top with roasted beets, goat cheese, and toasted walnuts.

- Drizzle with balsamic vinaigrette.

Cacao and Berry Smoothie

Ingredients:

- 1 cup mixed berries

- 1 tablespoon cacao powder

- 1/2 banana, frozen

- 1 cup almond milk

- 1 tablespoon chia seeds

Instructions:

- Blend berries, cacao powder, frozen banana, and almond milk until smooth.

- Stir in chia seeds and let it sit for a few minutes before consuming.

Spinach and Berry Salad with Citrus Dressing

Ingredients:

- 2 cups baby spinach
- 1/2 cup strawberries, sliced
- 1/4 cup blueberries
- 1/4 cup feta cheese, crumbled
- Citrus dressing

Instructions:

- Toss baby spinach with sliced strawberries, blueberries, and crumbled feta.
- Drizzle with citrus dressing.

Beetroot and Orange Smoothie

Ingredients:

* Beetroot (steamed or roasted)

* Oranges (peeled)

* Greek yogurt

* Honey

* Ice cubes

Instructions:

* Blend beetroot, oranges, Greek yogurt, and honey until smooth.

* Add ice cubes and blend again.

Garlic Lemon Salmon

73

Ingredients:

- Salmon fillets

- Garlic cloves (minced)

- Lemon juice

- Olive oil

- Fresh dill

- Salt and pepper

Instructions:

- Mix minced garlic, lemon juice, olive oil, fresh dill, salt, and pepper.

- Marinate salmon in the mixture for 30 minutes.

- Grill or bake until salmon is cooked.

THANKS   FOR

READING

THIS BOOK.